GOLF
AS GURU

GOLF
AS GURU

MINDFULLNESS, AWARENESS AND SELF-RESTRAINT

DR. JOHN EDWIN DEVORE

To order additional copies of this book, contact:
Xlibris
1-888-795-4274
www.Xlibris.com
Orders@Xlibris.com
801599

To Mom and Dad, my life's partners and caddies.

Contents

To find a man's true character, play golf with him.

—P.G. Wodehouse

Acknowledgments ix
Preface xi
Introduction xiii

Chapter 1   The Player and Integral Life Practice 1
Chapter 2   The Game 4
Chapter 3   Study, Reflection, and Practice 12
Chapter 4   Technical Skills 18
Chapter 5   Simply Golf 23
Chapter 6   Nineteenth Hole 30

Appendix A: Sample Vision, Current Reality Assessment, and Objectives 39
Appendix B: Left-Handed Golfer—Nine Ball-Flight Laws 41
Appendix C: Club Mechanics, Body Mechanics, Ball Positions,
             Routine, and Ritual 43
Appendix D: Green Reading and Putting Preshot Routine and Ritual 53
Resources 57
About the Author 63

ACKNOWLEDGMENTS

Many persons have pointed the way to joy that is happy independent of the need for what. Special thanks to Dad and Mom, my first golf partners. It was on December 1, 1948 that we launched the beginning of the golf journey. Dad wrote a check for one hundred dollars to purchase share #124 in the Buckeye Golf Club Company, doing business as Orchard Hills Country Club, Bryan, Ohio. I was eight years old. We took lessons from Shorty Stockman, head golf professional, and playing golf became a part of life then and now.

A particular note of thanks to son Doug—he wanted to learn to play golf in summer 2004. The first lesson with Doug at Indian Tree Golf Club, Arvada, Colorado, sparked my wife Cindy's interest in learning to play. She took lessons and has been a fearless, patient golf partner ever since. Daily, I am grateful for her wisdom, faith, hope, patience, and love. The kids—Doug, Debbie, and Chris—have offered priceless feedback, counsel, and guidance; and the six grandkids—Kelsie, TJ, Ivy, Jasmine, Calista, and Haley—are lights for the continued journey. Family is forever!

A final note of thanks is offered to the numerous authors who have contributed priceless efforts to my life because they have chosen to share their wisdom through published words.

PREFACE

Gowf is a mighty teacher never deviating from its sacred roots, always ready to lead us on...And I say to ye all, good friends, that as ye grow in gowf, ye come to see things ye learn in every other place...Ye'll come away from the links with a new hold on life, that is certain if ye play the game with all your heart.

—Michael Murphy

Golf is an evolving secret treasure of stories, legends, stellar global literature, and awareness experiences about the game and life. With mystical offerings and the prospect of tickled fantasies and inspired dreams, coupled with a plethora of life's priceless lessons and messages, a student of playing a ball with a club from the teeing ground into the hole by fewest successive strokes will quickly recognize that the impeccable journey of golf is the destination. This sport is a simple game, although difficult to play; and it is played on a field of friendly strife where peace can prevail or where mental and emotional chaos can emerge before every shot, during every shot, and between all shots. On any given day, the golfer is no less than two shanks, two slices, or two duck hooks from insanity. Fortunately, the ticket for release from this monkey mind, manufactured asylum is evolving *mindfulness, awareness,* and *self-restraint.* Marshall Gavre, a coach for Fred Shoemaker's Extraordinary Golf school, offers that the only difference between tour pros and us is that they are more aware during the two seconds it took to step up and swing.[1] Quite simply, golf "is nothing but a way or method to work on our inner or spiritual development. Through its teachings we try to change and transform the way we are, as well as the way we see ourselves and everything around us."[2]

As with other institutions, the art and science of playing a ball with a club has generated overwhelming volumes of "get it right" tips, systems, technologies, and instruction materials for all levels of golfers. As the seventy-plus years of golf

[1]   Extraordinary Golf: extragolf@aol.com. Fred Shoemaker publications: *Extraordinary Golf: The Art of the Possible* (1996). NY, NY: Perigee; and *Extraordinary Putting: Transforming the Whole Game* (2006). NY, NY: Perigee.

[2]   Tulku, 13.

and aging have evolved for the author, "simple, simple, simple" has become the screaming mantra; and a key learning is that as unique individuals we each need to find what works for us. As Arnold Palmer offered, "Swing your swing."

This offering is a heartfelt guide that can support the golfer who has clear goals and an authentic intent; and it has been created from personal experiences, literature, journals, after-round notes, and papers from academic work. Experience speaks loudly that to perform on-the-course, to enjoy the game, and to learn about the game requires an inquiring, curious, and open spirit, coupled with creativity and willingness to experiment, develop, and improve. As Tolstoy reminded, "The simplest thing cannot be made clear to the most intelligent man if he is firmly persuaded that he knows already, without a shadow of doubt, what is laid before him."[3]

Golf as Guru offers an Introduction that provides essential ingredients for "happy" golf. Chapter 1, "The Player and Integral Life Practice,"[4] embraces golf as a slice of life that can grow and awaken improved quality of life. Chapter 2, "The Game," offers a perspective of the game's components and sets the stage for Chapter 3, "Study, Reflection, and Practice." Chapter 4, "Technical Skills," outlines need-to-know basics for a decent round of golf; and Chapter 5, "Simply Golf," facilitates moving from goals and desires to playing golf. The "Nineteenth Hole" offers some conclusions and possible next steps.

The author's background, experiences, and interests can be found inside the back cover. As a committed student of golf, mindfulness, awareness, and self-restraint, you will soon recognize that the central message of this book is that awareness differentiates golfers and that good golf is playing and practicing a simple, synchronized inner and outer game. This sport demands absolute trust of the subconscious to create every shot by removing all except the supple human system, a club, a ball, and a target. This chosen sport is nothing more than clearing space for the artist within to sculpt a memorable shot. Bob Rotella offers, "Researchers have discovered that the body of a trained athlete has highly developed 'neural networks' that can subconsciously control the body's movements during execution of a complex athletic skill—like…pitching a golf ball off closely mowed grass, over a bunker, and onto a green so that it stops by the hole."[5]

---

[3] Christian and Tolstoy, 18.

[4] Ken Wilber's book, *Integral Life Practice: A 21st Century Blueprint for Physical Health, Emotional Balance, Mental Clarity, and Spiritual Awakening* delineates the concept of integral life practice. This concept is a way of organizing many life practices handed down through the centuries—along with cutting edge of psychology, consciousness studies, and other leading fields—using a framework optimized for life in the twenty-first century. It is ancient and modern, Eastern and Western, speculative and scientific, and foundational for evolving mindfulness, awareness, and self-restraint.

[5] Rotella, 61.

INTRODUCTION

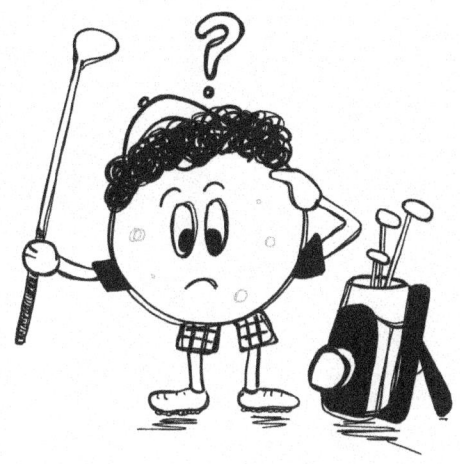

P laying "happy"[6] golf requires three swings: solid, centered impact, finesse swing, and putting stroke. It also has six games: putting, short game (chipping, pitching, and sand shots), scoring wedges (30-110 yards), power, body-mind, and on-the-course management.[7] The strategies of play are making and saving putts, hitting fairways, hitting greens in regulation, and making ups and downs. As a golfer's age and game evolve, a challenge is to have simple how-tos that facilitate enjoyment of play, quality practice, and growing awareness. Ingredients for ongoing contemplation about the game are as follows:

- The player and integral life practice
- The game
- Study, reflection, and practice
- Technical skills
- On-the-course management

---

[6] Joy is the result of happy that is not dependent on what happens.
[7] *Dave Pelz's Short Game Bible*, 32–43.

As play, enjoyment, and learning progress, inner awakening and outer growth evolve to become 80–90 percent of the game. The challenges are awakening and growing mindfulness, awareness, and self-restraint; learning to accept our human imperfections; and targeting for a perfect response on every shot. An evolving capacity to positively relate to experiences is critical to successes on-the-course and in life. Our gift of love to others is our wonderful smile that accompanies reflections in the world and golf shots as the course and each round unfold. Arnold Palmer offers a nice reminder, "The road to success is always under construction."[8]

---

[8]   Palmer, 52.

CHAPTER ONE

The Player and Integral Life Practice

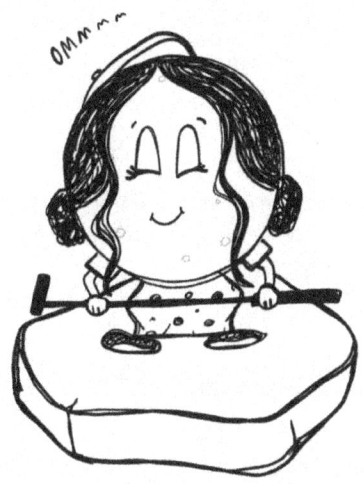

The Player

Player awareness[9]—of the self, life, and the game—differentiates golfers, evolves the "best of the best," and is the most important ingredient on every shot because of the need to juggle multitudes of environmental, technical, and human challenges. Of necessity are strategies that optimize human talents and skills with a goal of becoming one's best leader, manager, coach, teacher, caddie, and partner in life and golf. An inspiring way to develop and nurture the fullness of these opportunities is through study of the state-of-the-art integral theory work

---

[9]   Awareness—learning moved to experience and wisdom, consciousness, recognition, realization, and knowledge of a situation.

of Ken Wilber and the Integral Institute.[10] Integral theory is a comprehensive concept for exploring how humans show up in life—and golf—through four dimensions of being:

- *Individual interior:* Thoughts, feelings, intentions, and psychology.
- *Individual exterior:* Physical body and behavior.
- *Collective interior:* Culture, relationships, and shared meaning.
- *Collective exterior:* Institutions, environment, social structures, and systems.

Awakening and nurturing the development of these dimensions can result in liberation of unmanifested soul qualities; openness to true, naked reality by working with the body, mind, and spirit; and deeper psychological aspects of the human gift of life on and off-the-course. Our inner nature and the world beyond thought can truly begin to speak and to creatively be unleashed at will, on every shot. Yes! We can uncover processes that will help us quiet our monkey mind, reopen innate mindfulness and awareness, and enable learning self-restraint.

Integral Life Practice

> *Gently close your eyes and feel the sensations of the breath as the air passes the nostrils or upper lip. The sensations of the in-breath appear simply and naturally. Notice how the out-breath appears. Or you might choose to feel the movement of your chest or abdomen as the breath enters and leaves your body.*

—Joseph Goldstein

The gift of the human system is a remarkable treasure and invites utmost care if we are to live and play golf as well as we really can. As programmers of what we are, we are in a position to consider ideas for health, wellness and well-being, and the foundation of quality experiences in life and golf. Peter Jacobson remarks, "One of the most fascinating things about golf is how it reflects the cycle of life. No matter what you shoot, the next day you have to go back to the first tee and begin all over again and make yourself into something."[11]

The book *Integral Life Practice: A 21st-Century Blueprint for Physical Health, Emotional Balance, Mental Clarity, and Spiritual Awakening* is a practical, very flexible, awaiting guide for learning, and practicing how to awaken and grow to one's fullest capacities and perspectives in relationships, sport, career, parenting, communication, ethics

---

[10] Wilber, K. 2001. *A Brief History of Everything.* New York, NY: Penguin Random House. Wilber, K. 2001. *A Theory of Everything: An Integral Vision for Business, Politics, Science.* New York, NY: Penguin Random House.

[11] Hill, 141.

and morals, creativity, and life itself. With study, reflection, and practice the practitioner can (1) create a path to health, wellness, and well-being through the gross, subtle, and causal bodies; (2) nurture mental perspective and clarity for responses to reflections of the world; (3) use meditation to grow spaciousness for mental and emotional settling through becoming witness to personal reflections and triggers in the world; (4) dampen tortuous emotions and engage, take possession of, and integrate denied and repressed subconscious aspects of the self; (5) develop self-restraint and awaken and grow a compassionate ethical and moral foundation that thrives on love, kindness, hope, and affection; and (6) nurture pointers to silent self alone and a perfect response[12] to life's precious moments. Rabbi Zalman Schachter-Shalomi contends, "Integral Life Practice brings the integral system from the mind to doable action in life."[13] Quite simply, this is about physical exercise and peace of mind—cleaning up the hidden personal garbage and trapped emotions taken to every relationship, quieting the thinking mind and emotional reactions to free space for quality responses, and building a life of purpose on a foundation of morals, ethics, core values, guiding principles, and showing up for others. Wilber, Patten, Leonard, and Morelli suggest the following possibilities:[14]

- Embracing and working with crisis, pain, or suffering
- Becoming a better person on all levels, in all areas
- Living with integrity and excellence
- Getting over yourself
- Waking up
- As a way to understand everything or make sense of it all
- Living according to your highest levels
- Becoming more fully alive and creative
- Finding and/or living your deepest purpose
- Loving and caring for others more fully

Integral life practice, a living practice, "involves accepting all of life's textures, blessings and challenges as honored teachers…and viewing each life experience as a unique practice opportunity with a valuable lesson to bestow…Every now is a new practice opportunity."[15]

---

[12]   Cohen, 13-17.
[13]   Testimonial, *Integral Life Practice*, 2.
[14]   Wilber *et al*, 4.
[15]   Wilber *et al*, 287-88.

CHAPTER TWO

The Game

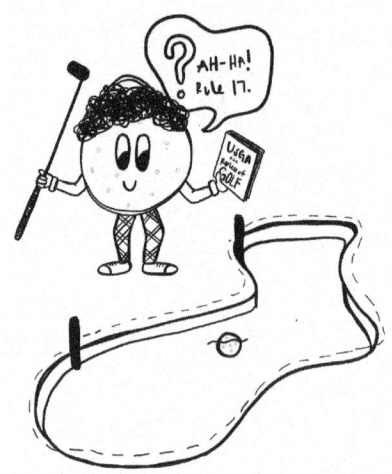

History

The history of the game is the foundation of its magnetic legacy. George Peper remarks in the *Story of Golf*, "No one can say precisely where or when the game of golf was born, but one thing is certain: No other form of recreation has transfixed its practitioners with such engaging appeal."[16]These first golf ancestors may have been Roman soldiers playing *paganica*, perhaps the Chinese during the Ming Dynasty, the English during the middle of the fourteenth century, or the French who played *jeu de mail* imported from Italy. The first written evidence was found at St. Andrews Links, Fife, Scotland, as early as 1552; and their first golf club was organized in 1754. The golf bug first hit America in 1888 when John

---

[16]   Peper, 13.

Reid, father of American golf, and five of his friends gathered in a pasture in Yonkers, New York, to have dialogue and give golf a try. The official beginning of golf in America was the founding of St. Andrews Golf Club, Yonkers, New York, on November 14, 1888.[17]

The sport of golf has been witness to (1) an evolution of equipment changes; (2) numerous success stories about professional golfers like Bobby Jones, Ben Hogan, Sam Snead, Jack Nicklaus, Arnold Palmer, Annika Sorenstam, Tiger Woods, Phil Mickelson, Jordan Speith, Justin Thomas, Dustin Johnson, *et al.*; (3) an overwhelming number of successful golf teaching professionals such as David Leadbetter, Joseph Parent, Butch Harmon, Jim McClean, Fred Shoemaker, and Todd Sones; and (4) a myriad of golf management and teaching professionals who have led and managed golf facilities and golf management companies around the world. A 2005 "Golf Economy Report"[18] indicated that the total economic impact of the golf industry in the United States was $195 billion, including 2 million jobs and $61 billion in wage income. The most recent international growth of golf is occurring in China and Eastern Europe. David De Nunzio, editor-in-chief, *Golf Magazine*, offers,

> In June (2019) the National Golf Foundation… released some promising participation numbers… 2.6 million represents the number of beginners who played on a course for the first time in 2018, a historic high…18 percent of these beginners were over the age of 50… the highest number in a decade. Unfortunately, junior participation sagged in 2018…18-34 year olds was stagnant … tech-driven outlets such as Top Golf ranges and full-swing simulator stores have helped spike interest in the game.[19]

Games within the Game

- Putting: putts up to six feet and lag putts
- Short game
  - Chipping and chi-putting[20]: normally up to 25 yards
  - Pitching: normally shots up to 30 yards, with spin and without spin
  - Sand shots: greenside and fairway sand bunkers
- Scoring wedges: 30-110 yards to hole
- Long game: 110 yards and longer to green

---

[17] Peper, 11–52.

[18] SRI International, commissioned by the leadership of Golf 20/20.

[19] *Golf Magazine*, "Welcome to the Machine," From the Editor, David De Nunzio, editor-in-chief, August 2019, 3.

[20] Pelz, D. 1999. See *Dave Pelz's Short Game Bible: Master the Finesse Swing and Lower Your Score*, New York, NY: Aurum, 219–220, 8.11 "The Chiputt."

- Body-mind mastery: physical, mental, and emotional skills
- On-the-course: synchronizing the inner and outer games, enjoying the walk, course strategizing, doing your best, and uncovering how good you are learning, practicing, and playing the game

Rules of Golf

Golf is played, for the most part, without the supervision of a referee or umpire. The game relies on the integrity of the individual to show consideration for other players and to abide by the Rules. All players should conduct themselves in a disciplined manner, demonstrating courtesy and sportsmanship at all times, irrespective of how competitive they may be. This is the spirit of the game of golf.[21]

Recommend becoming intimately familiar with (1) *Players Edition of the Rules of Golf*, (2) *Rules of Golf, Effective January* 2019, and (3) local rules for the golf course being played. All these rules are constantly changing and are updated periodically. The current *Rules of Golf* books can be purchased at www.usga.com or most golf equipment stores. Local rules are available in respective golf course pro shops. It is recommend that the current *Players Edition of the Rules of Golf* be kept in your golf bag. Both of the *Rules* books have rules of golf, pace-of-play guidelines, and definitions—the language of the game.

Etiquette and Behavior On-The-Course[22]

Practicing course etiquette respects the legendary core values and guiding principles of the game. Nothing is more frustrating than playing with a golfer who has not taken the time and opportunity to become familiar with course etiquette, the spirit of the game, safety, putting green courtesies, and mindful control of disturbance and distraction. Golf coaches, including my dad, always counseled as follows:

- Live the spirit of the game with integrity—be courteous and considerate of others, count all strokes, and play by the *Rules*. Unless stated in local rules or agreed to before teeing off on the first tee, players are not allowed to improve the lie of the ball on fairways or in roughs. You are on your honor to include penalties for grounding your club in sand traps and out of bounds, accidently moving the ball, and hitting another player's ball on the putting green.
- Prior to teeing off on the first tee: (1) discuss and agree on any special rules for this particular game—mulligans, strokes given or received, and

---

21   *Golf Rules Illustrated*, United States Golf Association, Hamlyn, 7.
22   *Ibid*, 7–8.

changing to a clean ball on the putting green and; (2) flip a coin or tee for honors on the first tee. Honors on subsequent tees go to the player with the lowest score on the hole just finished. In the event of a tie, honors revert to the winner of the preceding hole.

- Avoid standing close to or directly behind the ball when a player is about to play, and do not disturb play by fidgeting, moving, talking, or making unnecessary noise. Noisy electronic devices need to be shut off before arriving at the golf course.
- When a player drives a tee shot out of bounds, a nice gesture is to invite the player to take a short break, get composed, and not play another ball until other players have played. Play safe. Warn greens keeping staff who may be in danger and shout "fore" when there is danger of hitting someone. When other golfers are ahead of you, wait until they are one full shot ahead before you shoot.
- Repair divots on tees and in the fairway. A good practice is to use sand-seed mixture to repair divots on tees and fairways.
- Observe golf car movement signs.
- Always enter and leave sand traps on the low side. Rake footprints and sand divots in bunkers. Replace the rake in the bunker on the side away from the pin with the handle to tee.
- The player closest to the pin tends the flagstick for other players as they desire. The player whose ball is furthest from the hole putts or shoots first.
- On-the-green, when you are closer than other golfers, properly mark your ball with a golf ball marker. Players are on their honor to replace marked balls as precisely as possible. Loose impediments can be removed from your putting line, and fixing ball marks and green damage on the line of putt are permissible.
- Do not stand on another player's line of putt or directly behind the hole when he/she is making a stroke. When someone else is putting, other players should stand well out of his/her line of putt and field of vision; and these golfers should be aware of where their shadows are falling. Shadows should not be allowed to cross the putter's line of sight and, if possible, should be kept out of his/her peripheral view.
- Prevent unnecessary green damage. *Do not* drag, twist, or scuff your golf shoes. *Do not* place golf bags on-the-green. *Do not* pull golf carts on the green. *Do not* drive golf cars on the green. *Do not* stand too close to the hole. *Do not* use club heads to remove the ball from the hole, or lean on clubs on the green or when removing the ball from the cup. Repair green damage caused by golf shoes or ball marks with either a tee or divot tool. When removing the flag stick, carefully lay the pin on the fringe of the green.

- Wait on the green or green fringe until all players hole out and move away from the green as a group.
- Record scores on the way to the next hole.

Pace-of-Play

Slow play is the single most perplexing problem in the game of golf. A slow player can ruin the day for all players behind him/her. In the interest of all, players have an obligation to play at a reasonable pace. As an added variable in the pace-of-play equation, the number one revenue producer on golf courses is greens fees. Course management has an obligation to their respective boards or management teams to fill as many tee times with foursomes as are available. From this perspective, pace-of-play becomes a total team effort between golfers and course management. Some pace-of-play concepts to learn and practice are as follows:

-Play Ready Golf

- When you are ready to make the shot and it is safe, shoot.

-Courtesy

- Watch the shots of playing partners to facilitate locating golf balls for next shots.

-On-the-Tee

1. To facilitate ball identification, let other players know the name of the ball and the ball's markings you are playing.
2. Be ready to play when the fairway or green is clear.
3. Choose the set of tees that fits your game.
4. Shorter hitters should hit first.
5. Carry an extra ball in your pocket.
6. If it appears that your original ball may be difficult to find, it is a good idea to play a provisional ball.

-In the Fairway Rough

1. Hit when ready and safe.
2. Drop your cart partner off for their shot and drive to yours.
3. If another player is walking to their ball and you are ahead of them, make your shot.

4. Take multiple clubs to your ball and hit without delay.
5. Before reaching the green and having double par, pick up, place ball on green, and putt to hole out.

-On-the-Green

1. Before going to the green with your putter, golf cars, pull carts and carried golf club bags are positioned between the green on which you are going to putt and the next teeing ground.
2. First person on the green is in charge of tending the flag and watching for and retrieving clubs left on the green when leaving the green. When putting is complete, be ready to pick up and replace the flag. To prevent lost golf clubs, a good practice is to place the short game clubs you have used on the green between the flag and your golf car, golf cart, or golf bag.
3. Study and line up your putt while others are putting.
4. When practical, continue putting until holed out.
5. If a partner has a sand shot, be prepared to help with raking.
6. Leave the green immediately after holing out and proceed to the next tee.
7. Bag your clubs and complete your scorecard at the next teeing ground.

-On par 3 Greens

• Upon reaching the green, if the group behind you is waiting on the tee to hit, stand in a safe area and have the group hit.

-Water Balls

• If your ball goes into a water hazard and is accessible, take the time to retrieve only your ball.

-Lost Ball

• Limit search for lost balls to three minutes. If pressed for time and the next hole is open, wave the group behind through.

Be your own best pace-of-play coach by identifying the ways you can pick up the pace of play. *Rules of Golf,* Rule 5.6b, tells us, "When it is the player's turn to play:

• It is recommended that the player make the stroke in no more than 40 seconds after he or she is (or should be) able to play without interference or distraction, and

- The player should usually be able to play more quickly than that and is encouraged to do so."

Go to www.usga.com to learn about USGA pace-of-play programs, insights, and suggestions.

Equipment

Essential ingredients for good golf are a qualified club fitter and properly fitted and great-feeling equipment. As you reflect on putting together a game plan for equipment, consider the following:

- Enjoyment of the game is enhanced because properly fitted clubs just look, feel, perform, and sound good.
- With fitted clubs, the golfer has removed a key variable in the learning process.
- Save money! Do not shop for golf clubs unless you have your specifications in-hand and you know exactly what you intend to purchase. Golf club technology is a moving target, and marketers can reel you in very quickly with new head designs, grips, and shafts that are being mass produced and hitting the shelves every month. Normally, these manufacturers ship standard specifications with potentially wide manufacturing tolerances. Unfortunately, golf games are not improving, money is being wasted on equipment that does not meet advertised attributes, and more than likely, the newfangled club will not meet either your equipment specifications or perceived performance improvements.
- Experiment with different golf balls and consider being fitted for a golf ball that is matched to your club head speed.
- Good-fitting golf shoes that are broken in are a must. To facilitate breaking in new golf shoes, consider wearing them during your gym workouts.

Expect the following from a qualified and reputable club fitter:

1. A personal interview to determine what you are seeking in a new set of golf clubs; how you perceive the game; your skills, talents, strengths, and limitations; a budget for new equipment; and your golf goals and objectives.
2. Determine acceptable club head design in relation to your ability.
3. Establish proper length of clubs because it is the basis for consistency and accuracy.

4. Determine the proper lie for the clubs because it is a key for accuracy.
5. Establish the proper face angle because it is a critical variable for direction.
6. Establish necessary lofts, a variable that is key for trajectory and distance.
7. Determine the club shaft specifications: the shaft is the engine for the golf club and is critical for optimum distance and physical comfort for the golfer.
8. Determine optimum grip size because the grip establishes the relationship between the golfer's hands and the club.
9. Finally, optimize the weight of the golf club for optimum playability.

For those readers who are interested in further exploring the art of club fitting, I recommend *Total Clubfitting in the 21st Century: A Complete Program for Fitting Golf Equipment*(2007), Hierko Trading Company, Inc., 16185 Stephens Street, City of Industry, CA 91745, 800-367-8912.

CHAPTER THREE

Study, Reflection, and Practice

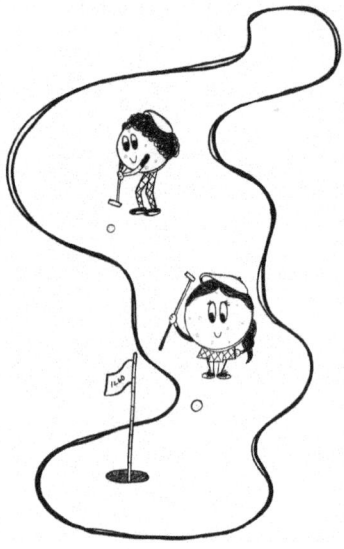

When we practice enough, we can sit back and enjoy the beauty of the process that flows through us. That is the process of being able to trust our abilities, which lies at the essence of being in the Zone.

—Michael Lardon

The challenges and opportunities for study, reflection, and practice of golf are many. In *The Inner Game of Golf,* Tim Gallwey offers,

Golf has an uncanny way of endearing itself to us while at the same time evoking every weakness of mind and character, no matter how well hidden. The common purpose served is that we either learn to overcome the weaknesses or we are overwhelmed by them. Few games provide such an ideal arena for confronting the very obstacles that impair one's ability to learn, perform and enjoy life, whether on or off the golf course. But to take advantage of this opportunity, the golfer must accept the challenge to play the Inner Game as well as the Outer Game.[23]

Rosemary Fuchs contends, "Practice is not a fixed entity. It includes anything that helps us to improve our attitude and to gain authentic experiential understanding of the true nature of everything. We are our practice and the only measure is our own spiritual development."[24] Quite simply, golf can become a spiritual awareness growing experience. To inspire nurturing awareness, let's explore learning types, learning principles, neuroscience, and instructors.

Learning Types

Juggling the multitude of inner and outer skills requires that one constantly remind the inner roommate—the pesky, self-serving ego-mind—that the goal is to study, to reflect, to evolve awareness, to practice, and to play *your* game. A necessary strategy is to be curious, to experiment, and to uncover your most effective and efficient learning and practicing style or styles. For reflection and discovery, some learning types and explanations[25] are as follows:

- *Verbal or auditory.* The input for the human system is hearing. These individuals like to write down what they have heard and frequently repeat statements to make sure they have heard correctly.
- *Visual.* The input for the human system is seeing. These individuals like pictures, videos, and demonstrations, and they focus on details of body and club mechanics.
- *Kinesthetic.* The input for the individual is feeling based on awareness of the human system. They need to perform the physical, mental, and emotional activity. They normally have a high degree of hand-eye coordination, are accomplished athletes, and use recall of body mechanics for subconscious programming.

---

23   Gallwey, 8.
24   Tulku, 9.
25   *Golf Academy of America Teaching Manual, 2nd edition* (2009), Chapter 3, 31–34.

- *Innovative.* The input for the human system is personal experience to make sense of new materials. They have a strong need to know why the new information is useful.
- *Analytical.* These individuals have a need to know what and why the new material is important. They are normally good listeners.
- *Common sense.* These folks want action and not talk.
- *Dynamic.* All these individuals need is conceptual guidance before being turned loose to add personal experience to any project encountered.
- *Contemplation.*[26] The process of receiving information, perking that information, and experiencing the information. First, we gather an intellectual understanding by receiving information, or knowledge, through the senses of hearing, seeing, or reading. This information is then perked: we reflect on the content of the information and ponder how our human system feels about this new knowledge. Does the new material fit our human system? A final step is an activity, a vehicle for transformation or a practice, like meditation for quieting, concentrating, and focusing the mind. This final step is to dwell in silence and solitude with the new information to gather personal insight and experience the Self in action. This final step has the potential to move knowledge to experience and wisdom.
- *Awareness.*[27] What the human system is experiencing in the moment. His Holiness the Dalai Lama states,

> Awareness…means paying attention to our own behavior. It means honestly observing our behavior as it is going on, and thereby bringing it under control. By being aware of our words and actions, we guard ourselves against doing and saying things we will later regret. When we are angry, for instance, and if we fail to recognize that our anger is distorting our perception, we may say things we do not mean. So having the ability to monitor oneself, having, as it were, a second order level of attention, is of great practical use in everyday life, as it gives us greater control over our negative behavior and enables us to remain true to our deeper motives and convictions.[28]

Yes! If we are open to it, golf can be a guru. Mindfulness, awakening, and growing awareness and learning self-restraint are the primary faculties we have for knowing and learning from experience, integrating body-mind mastery and technical skills, and closely replicating play on-the-course. Our sensual experiences are the language of the neural system that programs the muscles to

---

[26]   Naropa University learning modality.

[27]   See Shoemaker, F. 1996. *Extraordinary Golf: The Art of the Possible.*

[28]   Dalai Lama, 109.

provide the body mechanics that optimize club to ball contact at impact. The muscles and the mind do not speak the same language. As a result, the mind is not able to tell the muscles what to do. We need to learn that the mind is a tool to help us learn to program the subconscious to perform; however, when it comes to performance, one must quiet the mind and trust the subconscious to perform— breathe deep, ground the physical system, heighten the emotions, focus attention, quiet the mind, and pull the trigger. More often than not, thinking gets in our way and becomes an obstacle to optimum performance on and off the golf course.

This concept of awareness is nothing more than being a silent watcher of sensual inputs, thoughts, emotions, and physical sensations. The sensual inputs are processed through touching, seeing, hearing, tasting, and smelling. Thoughts originate in the mind, emotions are associated with thoughts and are experienced in the body, and physical sensations are felt in the body. If the golfer wants to change something, a first step is to increase awareness of the way it is. Just focus on a specific area and become more aware of what is there. It is always a nice thought that there are many times when our human system gets it right by not even trying. After focused awareness, there are many times when the human system will simply self-correct. Some examples with which to experiment are the following:

1. What does a golfer feel during the swing of a golf club? Feel the turning club head during takeaway. Feel the hurried transition at top of backswing. Feel the shape of the swing plane—flat, vertical, jerky, or smooth?

2. What is happening with clubface angle at impact—open, closed, or square? Experiment with clubface angle by trusting the subconscious to either open, close, or square the clubface at impact. Recall that the keys are to acknowledge reflections in the world (what is manifesting in the mind), to remain open to receive messages, to ponder the inputs, and to trust the subconscious to get the job done.

Learning Principles and Neuroscience

In *The Adult Learner*, Knowles, Holton, and Swanson discuss the learning needs of adults and the impact of neuroscience on learning.

• We need to know the *what*, *how*, and *why* of the subject matter being learned.
• We are self-directed learners because our capability has been demonstrated through past successes.

- Experience is the foundation for our new learning. New information is processed using existing networks built from prior learning, experiences, background, and interests.
- We are ready to learn because we have identified the self-actualization need.
- Our evolved conscious and subconscious interference may be an obstacle because the subject to be learned will not solve life's problems or is not on the to-do list. Obstacles are inner-roommate interference—people, places, events, complexity, and lists, and more lists. The self is a simple sentinel when the world behaves, and one needs to acknowledge reflections in the world because the Self is the reflections. As Tolstoy writes in his diary, "It's impossible to describe a man (people, places, and/or events) but it is possible to describe the effect he (they) has (have) on me."[29]
- We need a clear motivation to learn.

Brain research offers that learning desired change is enabled by changing the way synapses communicate with one another via neurotransmitters. Positive emotions generate increased neurotransmitters, stimulate learning, generate satisfaction, and increase motivation. Negative emotions stagnate learning. Four adult practice guidelines are as follows:

- Daily, practice consistently at the same time for at least fifteen minutes.
- Pay attention to details. Practice sessions need specific tasks and a time for each task.
- Practice the tasks enjoyed.
- Practice the way you learn best.

Instructors

An instructor needs to become aware, understand, and commit to a process that facilitates a student's learning. A student's self-awareness of how they best learn can certainly help the instructor optimize instructor-student time together. Awareness and contemplation have evolved to be my superior learning modalities. As a result, a preference is for a good coach. Teachers tell you what they like to have you do—their system. Coaches will uncover what your desires are and help you get there.

Needless to say, golf has a bunch of stuff to study, reflect upon, practice, and learn. Practice enables us to harmonize and integrate brain stuff in order to respond to the inevitable challenges of life and golf with a quiet mind, less

---

[29]   Christian and Tolstoy, 56.

fragmentation, and more integration—less fear, anger, and sadness and more peace, happiness, and joy. We can google information in seconds, but real knowledge and wisdom take time. Just enjoy the journey and taste the spiritual sweets—the tingling, calming, concentration ritual before the next shot. Dan Millman contends,

> Masters of one art have mastered the inner principles of all arts because they have mastered themselves. With dominion over both mind and muscle, they demonstrate power, serenity, and spirit. They not only have talent for sport, they have an expanded capacity for life. The experts shine in the competitive arena; the masters shine everywhere.[30]

Whatever you are practicing, always reserve silent moments to celebrate and experience expanding awareness. Awareness differentiates golfers, and it is the key to our protection—like sunscreen—against the interference and snares from monkey mind attachments and aversions.

---

[30] Millman, 168.

CHAPTER FOUR

Technical Skills

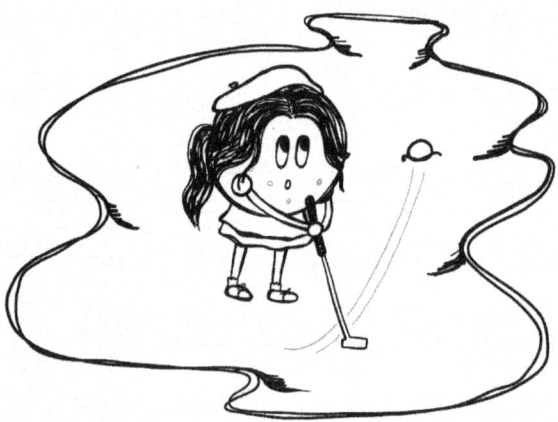

The intent of this chapter is to offer technical fundamentals that can create a foundation on which a golfer might be inspired to grow and nurture awareness, to become a true student of the game, to practice more effectively and efficiently, to perform better on-the-course, and to enhance enjoyment of the game.

Logistical Factors

The two logistical factors that require consideration on each shot are *direction* and *distance*. Direction concerns right or left accuracy of shots or how far left or right of target the ball is or will be. Distance concerns how far the golf ball has traveled or how long or short the ball will be in relation to the chosen target.

Ball Flight Laws

There are five ball flight laws that control a ball's flight. These laws need to be studied, learned, and managed. With focused practice, these laws can grow awareness of the golf swing.

- Clubface angle
- Clubface path
- Angle of the club's approach to the ball
- Centeredness of impact of the ball with the clubface
- Speed of the clubface at impact

The two primary variables that control ball flight direction are clubface angle and clubface path. Trackman data indicate that for <u>irons</u> **clubface angle** at impact controls **75%** of ball flight direction; and that **clubface path** at impact controls **25%** of ball flight direction. For the <u>driver</u> Trackman data indicate that **clubface angle** at impact controls **85%** of ball flight direction; and that **clubface path** at impact controls **15%** of ball flight direction.

The clubface path at impact dictates the initial ball flight direction. Its path can be inside-out, straight, or outside-in to the ball-target line. The clubface angle at impact dictates the secondary ball flight direction. This angle can be closed, square, or open to the ball-target line. Together, the clubface angle and clubface path result in nine different ball flights that can be read and managed.

Right-Handed Golfer
(Note: if you are a lefty, see Appendix B: Left-Handed Golfer—Nine Ball-Flight Laws.)

1. *Push-draw* (inside-out, clubface closed). The ball flies straight but to right of target and then bends-draws-hooks[31] to the left.
2. *Push* (inside-out, clubface square). The ball flies straight but to right of target.
3. *Push-fade* (inside-out, clubface open). The ball flies straight but to right of target and then bends-fades-slices[32] to right.

---

[31] Hook—for right-handed golfer ball starts right of target then bends rather *sharply* to the left; for left handed golfer ball starts left of target then bends rather *sharply* to the right.

[32] *Slice.* For a right-handed golfer, the ball starts left of target then bends rather *sharply* to right; for a left-handed golfer, the ball starts right of target then bends rather *sharply* to left.

4.   *Straight-draw* (straight, clubface closed). The ball flies straight and then bends-draws-hooks left

5.   *Straight* (straight, clubface square). The ball is on target.

6.   *Straight-fade* (straight, clubface open). The ball flies straight and then bends-fades-slices right.

7.   *Pull-draw* (outside-in, clubface closed). The ball flies straight but to left of target and then bends-draws-hooks left.

8.   *Pull* (outside-in, clubface square). The ball flies straight but to left of target.

9.   *Pull-fade* (outside-in, clubface open). The ball flies straight but left of target and then bends-fades-slices right.

Fourteen Principles

The fourteen principles are mechanical elements of the golf swing and can help solve distance and direction issues. They are factors that have a direct relation to and significant influence on the laws but require a certain amount of golfer or instructor awareness and subjective judgment with respect to application about mechanics of the swing for individual golfers.

When ball flight is incorrect, it most likely was a result of poor set-up because for the driver it is normally the cause of 85 percent of errant ball flight effects (75 percent for irons). When working with club mechanics and body mechanics, a properly selected principle is most probably the root cause of a ball flight effect. Example: the distance can be reduced when the left arm of a right-handed golfer is bent on takeaway and forward swing because the width of arc of the arms and club is less than optimum, resulting in less than optimum centrifugal force of the club head on impact with the ball. The fourteen principles—with respective direction, distance, or direction-distance impact—are as follows:

Direction Influence

- *Grip.* The placement of the hands on the golf club. It is the connection of the golfer to the golf club. The grip is open, closed, or neutral.
- *Aim.* Alignments of the clubface and body—feet, hips, and shoulders—in relation to the target.
- *Position.* Relationship of the back of the leading forearm, wrist, and hand at the top of the back swing. The wrist is flat, cupped, or arched.
- *Swing plane.* A pane of glass that matches the path of the club shaft; the tilt and direction of travel of the inclined plane that is made by the club shaft as it moves through the backswing and the downswing.
- *Release.* Return of the body, arms, and club head to a position that is similar to their starting position. This allows energy that was created

during the back swing to be released through the club head to the ball at impact.

Distance Influence

- *Width of arc.* Amount of extension of golfer's hands away from the swing center during the swing.
- *Length of arc.* Total distance the club head travels during the back swing and forward swing.
- *Lever system.* Levers formed by the lead arm and the club during the back swing; hinging the wrists and positioning the club shaft approximately 90 degrees to the leading arm; wrist cocking occurs on the backswing and uncocking release occurs on the forward swing.

Distance and Direction Influence

- *Connection.* Positioning and maintaining the various body parts in relation to one another in set-up and during the swing, maintaining the club, grip, right shoulder and left shoulder triangle and parts working together. Connection is critical during transition from back swing to forward swing.
- *Set-up.* Combination of foot placement, ball positioning, body posture, muscular readiness, and weight distribution.
- *Timing.* Combined sequence of movement of the body and the club to produce efficient, synchronized body mechanics and club mechanics.
- *Swing center.* Point between the top of the spine on the back of the body and the top of the sternum on the front of the body.
- *Dynamic balance.* Maintaining body control during the swing as the golfer transfers weight from the trailing foot to the leading foot and from the leading foot to the trailing foot. The ability to maintain balance while in motion is essential before learning other direction principles.
- *Impact.* Moment of truth; striking through the ball with the center of the clubface with as few compensating moves as possible.

In addition to ball flight laws and swing principles, a term discussed is *preferences.* Preferences constitute a third level of priorities in establishing a golf swing, yet they are important because it is at this level that we most often practice and play. A preference is the act of choosing or liking better some particular approach, method, device, etc. over all others. Examples of chipping preferences: ball position even with the inside of the heel of the right foot; stance open with both feet; ball position either forward off front foot (high trajectory) or off the trailing foot (low trajectory); hinge and hold chip or stable wrist chip. Examples of pitching preferences: ball played from center of stance; ball played from forward in stance (high trajectory) or center of stance (low trajectory).

The intent of this chapter has been to offer basic, technical fundamentals that can nurture and grow awareness of how best to optimize practice and play. As your game progresses, you may find that Appendix C: Club Mechanics, Body Mechanics, Ball Position, Routine, and Ritual will offer additional technical skills for the shots of the game: putting, chipping, pitching, sand shots, scoring wedges, and long game. Enjoy this beautiful, evolving awareness journey to uncover your best!

CHAPTER FIVE

Simply Golf

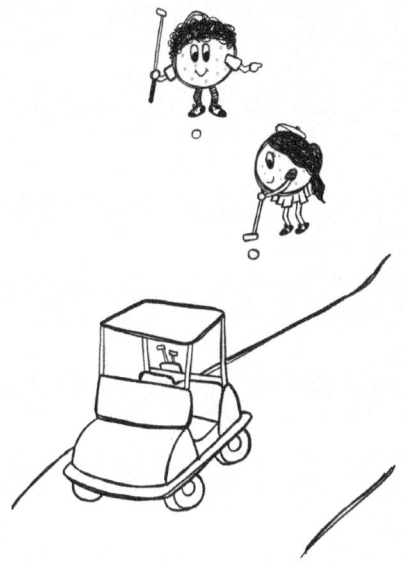

Golf is deceptively simple and endlessly complicated.

—Arnold Palmer

A typical golf shot cycle consists of five elements: warm-up, preparation, action, response, and recovery.

Warm-up

Warm-up includes the psychological and behavioral processes that golfers go through before beginning a round of golf and before every shot during a round of golf. In *The Game Before the Game*, Lynn Marriot and Pia Nilsson contend, "A thoughtful transition from the chaos around us to the calm within is necessary to play good golf."[33] To stimulate pre-round and warm-up creative juices, consider the following:

- Warm up the physical body with a few stretching exercises.
- Hit a few balls with two-three clubs.
- Deep breathing for tension relief and transition.
- Sit, be silent, and enjoy the solitude of being with nature and friends.
- Make a few chips, pitches, and putts.
- If necessary, decide on a swing thought for the round.
- Take a few rehearsal swings to facilitate feel for tempo, rhythm, and timing.

Coop and Wiren contend,

The state of the body can influence the mood of the mind…in three ways…

1. Through a pre-round routine of warm-up drills, which helps the body make the transition from off-course activities to actual play more smoothly.
2. Through a fixed pre-shot routine, which keeps the body in a more relaxed state before every shot.
3. Through a rehearsal-swing routine, which helps the body stay relaxed on short shots and trouble shots that are intrinsically more anxiety producing.[34]

Preparation

Preshot Routine[35]

---

[33]   Marriott and Nilsson, 16.

[34]   Coop and Wiren, 156.

[35]   Design preshot routines that work for you. This routine is offered as only input. For green reading, putting preshot routine and putting ritual, see Appendix D: Green Reading and Putting Preshot Routine and Ritual. The green information is a personal golf cart checklist created from *Dave Pelz's Putting Bible*. 2020. New York, NY: Doubleday.

The preshot routine ensures that the goal of every shot is crystal clear and that the motivation is created to sustain the desired result. The typical golfer wants preshot routines to be the same for each type of shot from one shot to the next, and each time you go through the routine, you want it to take approximately the same amount of time.

The tools one has to create a solid, consistent routine are attention and intention. Attention is the tool of the mental body and is the *what* of our focus—single-pointed attention on the visual picture of the synchronized physical body swinging a club and a ball at impact being sweetly struck and moved beautifully to a precise target. Intention is the tool of the emotional body and is the *why* of our focus. Five, short, explosive breaths into the upper chest to activate the sympathetic nervous system increase oxygen and intensify subtle energy currents preparing the whole body for the exertion to come. The quality of each shot experience is determined by how consciously attention and intention are wielded. The challenge is to be present to consciously use these tools to serve us physically, emotionally, and mentally for every shot—ground the physical body, elevate the emotional body, and focus the mind.

After typical shot preliminaries—relaxation techniques, target selection, checking the lie of the ball, planning strategies for wind direction and strength, estimating distance, and making the club selection—a sample preshot routine might look as follows:

1. Stand behind the ball on the ball-target line and make practice strokes to clear a busy mind and subconsciously program the swing necessary to move the ball to the target.
2. Walk to the ball along the ball-target line mentally embracing the club, the optimum swing, the target, and the ball arriving on target.
3. Go to the breath to activate awareness. Focus on the in-out breath and begin to quiet the mind, release tension, and create space for awareness. Swing thoughts evolve to become only passing thoughts. As deliberate, deep breathing continues, the golfer is focused.
    ➤ *Grip.* Hands act as a single unit, not too loose and not too tight.
    ➤ *Aim.* Parallel flow lines[36] of feet, knees, hips, forearms, and shoulders are aligned parallel with ball-target line.
    ➤ *Set up.* Fine-tune ball position, stance, and posture. Square the clubface and dance to feel static and dynamic balance. You are now ready for action with your unique ritual.

---

[36] Pelz, 100.

Action

Ritual

A good athlete can enter a state of body awareness in which the right stroke or the right movement happens by itself effortlessly without any interference of the conscious will. This is the paradigm for non-action, the purest and most effective form of action. The game plays the game; the poem writes the poem; we can't tell the dancer from the dance.[37]

For every shot, the golfer needs to evolve a ritual for creating a personal teepee where the mind becomes clear and quiet[38] and the physically and mentally programmed subconscious is given absolute trust to deliver a shot. In 1929, legendary Bobby Jones remarked,

> The golf swing is a most complicated combination of muscular actions, too complex to be controlled by objective conscious mental effort. Consequently, we must rely a good deal upon the instinctive reactions acquired by long practice. It has been my experience that the more completely we can depend upon this instinct—the more thoroughly we can divest the subjective mind of conscious control, the more exclusion of all thoughts as to method—is the secret of a good shot...After taking the stance, it is too late to worry. The only thing to do is to hit the ball.[39]

It could be argued that pulling the trigger to make the shot is the most critical of all elements of the shot cycle, and it may be the simplest and yet possibly the most difficult because it must be done without thinking and with <u>absolute trust of the subconscious</u> to perform to expectations. As we settle to create the space bubble—the state of relaxed concentration—we are deliberately breathing. The ritual is automatic and is the one distinct stimulus that will trigger and coordinate all the elements that facilitate emergence of the peak performance state. We are empty and the trigger is absently pulled.

This evolving master skill is individually unique and is the state of being present, tension-free, with that which is intended for as long as intended.[40] Summon the inner artist for a remarkable and often indescribable zone experience of spiritual oneness; and be witness to freedom and an intuitive unleashing of a

---

[37]   Mitchell, S. 2006. *Tao te ching*. New York, NY: Harper, viii.

[38]   Shoemaker uses "clear and quiet state-of-mind" in *Extraordinary Golf*. This concept has also been referred to as relaxed concentration (Gallwey) and flow state (Csikszentmihalyi).

[39]   Gallwey, 19–20.

[40]   Shoemaker, *Extraordinary Putting*, 8–10.

unique, creative, synchronous flow of human physical activity. Simply relax and put your awareness where your deepest natural breathing originates—sensed image approximately 1½ inches below your navel. Let breathing be deep and full, shake loose any tension in the muscles, and trust that as center is experienced, there is seamless unity of body, mind, and spirit, setting the stage for "sweet impact" and zone performance. Well-practiced actions will result naturally without effort. A quick and dirty master's ritual checklist for every shot must include the following:

- *Ground.* Take a couple of deep breaths and visualize energy circulating between your feet and the earth below you. Feel static and dynamic balance and sense a balanced, solid foundation and the environment surrounding you.
- *Elevate.* Take three to five short, explosive breaths into the upper chest to activate the sympathetic nervous system, increase oxygen, and intensify subtle energy currents. Charge the whole body, physically and emotionally, preparing for the exertion to come. Make a final visual touch of the target and smile.
- *Relaxed focus.* On an out-breath, one-pointed concentration on the point of impact of club with ball (mindfulness), channeling all body energies into a laser beam of relaxed, focused concentration, letting go of everything (self-restraint), and sensing the synchronous, flowing swing to impact with a ball creatively floating to the target (awareness).

Squeeze Trigger: With passion burning, the captain of the ship squeezes the auto-pilot button and trusts the programmed subconscious to creatively deliver a ball to an intended target.

Recovery

Recovery restores health to the human system and can include responding, learning, relaxing, and preliminary thoughts about the next shot. *I am centered, calm, silent, present, and at peace. My choice is to experience this moment.* Smell the roses, enjoy the day, take a deep breath, smile—our gift of love to others—and be at peace. As the period of recovery nears its end, it includes, of necessity, transitioning the body-mind for that next encounter with the new canvas, your artist's tools, a golf ball, and the associated challenges of the next shot and the next moment. Every moment of life has a purpose that one can choose to embrace and energize; and in the present moment, one enjoys life and golf saturated with meaning.[41] Simply, life punctuated with simple golf.

Responding

---

[41]   Brown, 144.

"Yes! Wow! Great shot!" Responding is emotional—the Tiger Woods, Phil Mickelson, Dustin Johnson, and Rory McIlroy fists and arm pumps when they sink those necessary, critical putts on eighteenth greens to win $1.5 million. This is openly acknowledging the thrill and excitement of watching the beauty of a ball's trajectory; hearing the sound of the club and ball at impact; or seeing the ball hit the green, bounce, and come to rest near the pin. This is celebrating the bunker shot that leaves a four-foot putt, and this is jumping into the air and letting the world know you just made that first hole in one.

Needless to say, responding to the experience of a golf shot can create the need to manage negative emotions (self-restraint), too. An errant golf shot is a fine opportunity—and challenge—to acknowledge our reflections in the world and learn from them. These errant shots can help one surface and integrate heretofore subconscious behaviors and certainly can support learning to dampen the detrimental impact that the dreaded demon of tension can have on our golf game. If we remain open, these challenges can offer improvement messages and support our efforts to study, reflect upon, and practice specific elements of the game. Concerning response to good shots, Coop and Wiren offer,

> Psychologist Peter Cranford draws the analogy that a good round of golf is a string of pearls. Each shot is a precious pearl that takes your full attention to create. You can only create one at a time, so don't concern yourself with those you have already made or those you have yet to make. Focusing on adding one pearl, individually, leads to the creation of a fine finished product.[42]

Learning

How did the preshot routine and ritual processes work? What needs practice? What needs coaching? What additional skills will support development and reduction of interference? How are the clubs working? How do the shoes feel? Collecting key, on-the-course data may support spending practice time on what counts for progress in your game. Some player development data you may find helpful to collect and study are as follows:

- Fairways hit
- Fairways missed and whether missed left or right
- Greens hit in regulation
- Greens missed in regulation and whether missed short, long, left, or right
- Ups and downs made
- Ups and downs missed and why—putt, chip, pitch, etc.

---

[42]   Coop and Wiren, 114.

- Number of putts
- Score
- Penalty shots

Relaxing

Focus on deep breathing while counting the out breaths. Count to ten and reverse the count to zero. Just let go and be free—*I am the silent self alone. It has been a wonderful day. I am grateful and the big smile beams of hope, faith, and love. Life is great!*

CHAPTER SIX

Nineteenth Hole

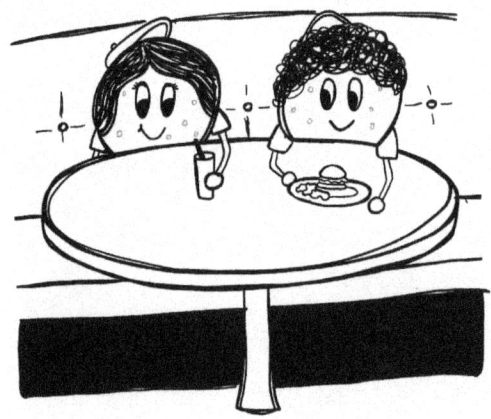

The most rewarding things you do in life are often the ones that look like they cannot be done.

—Arnold Palmer

The "Nineteenth Hole" offers a touch of philosophy and bucket lists that can be helpful for study, reflection, practice, and improvement. Growing and nurturing mindfulness, awareness, and self-restraint are an evolving and rewarding journey. Celebrate your gift of life and have fun!

The Player

- Tap into Andrew Cohen's theory and journey—the art and science of stillness, clarity of intention, the power of volition, face everything and avoid nothing, the process perspective, and cosmic conscience.[43]
- Commit to the concept that awareness—of the Self and the game—differentiates golfers. Who am I? What is this game of golf about? How can I create a wedding between this student and the game?
- Know why you play the game, and focus on playing the game to satisfy that purpose.
- Become your best leader, manager, coach, teacher, caddie, and partner when studying, practicing, and playing.
- Evolve a go-to refocusing formula[44] to use on-the-course when the wheels have fallen off the game and insanity looms.
- Nurture insatiable curiosity and openness about the Self and the game. Simply understand why that does *that* and how to create *that* at will.
- Grow the capacity to ignite passion and to create space for zone performance on every shot.
- Create a golf vision, annually assess current reality, and prepare measureable short-term objectives that will help close the vision-current reality gap. See Appendix A: Sample Vision, Current Reality Assessment, and Objectives.

Integral Life Practice

- Remain as physically and mentally active as possible. Create a physical exercise program; have quality relationships with family, friends, and community; practice mental well-being through stress control at will; eat healthy foods; get enough rest and adequate sleep at night; and actively manage and participate in your healthcare decisions.[45]

---

[43] Cohen, A. 2011. *Evolutionary Enlightenment: A New Path to Spiritual Awakening.* New York, NY: Select Books.

[44] Example formula: go to the breath; *acknowledge* the unhealthy, ego mind talk; *decide* the interference is detrimental to full potential; *send* the ego mind, interfering chatter packing; and in silence, *mindfully create space and conditions* for conscious free will to awaken and zone performance to manifest.

[45] *Health Smarts: Tips for happy healthy Superagers* (Summer 2018). Banner Health Network, "Doc TALK," page 4.

- Become a body-mind master. Create an integral life practice[46] program for physical health, emotional balance, mental clarity, and spiritual awakening.
- Recommend locating a meditation instructor and learning mindfulness and awareness meditation. Meditation will not fix anything; however, it exposes habitual patterns which obstruct awareness and present moment focus. Some of the skills that can evolve are as follows:

  ✓ Connected breath that facilitates relaxation as one prepares to begin the preshot routine.
  ✓ A growing capacity to declutter and open the mind, create an environment of less stress, and enable accomplishing more than previously.
  ✓ Evolving ability to create a heartfelt visualization of the desired shot.
  ✓ Relaxed concentration at will to enable trust of the subconscious as one squeezes the trigger.
  ✓ Enhanced optimum flow and power of the relaxed, supple body at point of impact of the clubface moving through the ball to the target.
  ✓ An authentically joyful response to the beauty of the sculpted shot.
  ✓ On-the-course and off-the-course—insight into the ego mind, its conditioned concepts and beliefs and associated behaviors that manifest through body, speech, and mind.
  ✓ One can learn to be a mind watcher and uncover an ability to listen to the chatter of the pesky inner roommate.

Thich Nhat Hanh notes,

> Once you've learned how to stop your mind when your body is also stopped, you'll be able to stop your mind even when your body is moving.[47] You use your mindfulness to become aware of everything, of every feeling, every perception in yourself, as well as what's happening around you...[48]

Andrew Cohen offers,

---

[46] See Wilber, K. *et al.* 2008. *Integral Life Practice: A 21st Century Blueprint for Physical Health, Emotional Balance, Mental Clarity, and Spiritual Awakening.* Boston, MA: Integral.

[47] Thich Nhat Hanh, 64.

[48] *Ibid*, 151.

Meditation is that state of consciousness that reveals itself when we take no position in relation to thought. When we take no position in relationship to thought, the whole world and everything in it, including our own mind, falls away from us. Our experience is one of ecstatic freedom from boundaries, of finding ourselves blissfully alone, happily lost deep in the unknown. And if we can continue to resist the temptation to take any position in relationship to arising of thought, we will find ourselves in a place that is impossible to describe in words. A place that is completely free. It is a place of perfect fullness and perfect stillness. It is a place where nothing ever happened.[49] When you meditate, you consciously choose to assume the enlightened relationship to your own experience, which means you are *letting everything go*...Meditation, as a metaphor for enlightenment, is the practice of the unconditional willingness to be free from, to transcend, and to let go of anything in your way.[50]

- Practice sensing static balance and dynamic centering, "the highest degree of mobility with a center which remains immovable."[51]
- Master creating your ritual and relaxed concentration teepee[52] for every shot.
- Create a solid foundation of ethics, morals, values, and guiding principles and modeling the way as a person, in relationships, and by helping and supporting others.
- Commit to accept 100 percent responsibility—*Life happens because of me and not to me.*
- Nurture, awaken, and grow your creativity and uncover unmanifested soul qualities.

---

49 Cohen, *Living Enlightenment*, 103.

50 Cohen, *Evolutionary Enlightenment*, 102–103.

51 Crum, 114.

52 Gallwey, "Relaxed Concentration: The Master Skill," 169–185; Shoemaker, "Concentration," 50–60, 195–96. Conceptualize that the human mind has an "inner roommate" who pesters and a "watcher" who is the sentinel: in a state of relaxed concentration the "inner roommate" is absent and the "watcher" is present and abiding. As used in this book, this is the natural state of the subconscious. As golfers, it is important to grasp that concentration of thought cannot occur unless the "watcher" has learned and practiced guiding the flow of thought, taming the monkey mind, and quieting the patterns of interference.

The Game

- Know history, etiquette, pace-of-play guidelines, and the *Rules of Golf.*
- Have proper equipment and equipment that fits, looks good, and feels good.
- Master the games in the game—putting, short game, scoring wedges, power, mental, and course management.

Study, Reflection, and Practice

- Know learning style or styles and how best to study, reflect, and practice.
- Grasp the unique nature of the concept of awareness—if something needs to change, it will change as we increase awareness of it.
- Interview and select a good coach.
- At the right time, arrange to take a playing lesson with your coach. Prior to the scheduled date of the lesson, meet with the coach to complete a shot-cycle game plan (i.e. discuss and agree on specific roles, focus, and objectives for the playing lesson). On the scheduled date of the lesson, learn on-the-course with the shot-cycle game plan.
- Priorities for practice: (1) putting (lag putts and putts less than six feet), (2) short game (chipping, pitching, and sand shots), (3) scoring wedges (distances and accuracy), and (4) long clubs.

Technical Skills

- *Create key elements for each of your shots.* Categories for key elements are body mechanics, club mechanics, ball position, routine, and ritual. See Appendix C: Club Mechanics, Body Mechanics, Ball Positions, Routine, and Ritual.
- *Impeccable set-up* (GASP, as in "grip, aim, stance, and posture"). The set-up is 80–85 percent of a good swing.
- *Master one piece takeaway.* The club, hands, and arms move as a single unit. You are now at 90-95 percent of a good swing.
- *Stable right side* (LH golfers, stable left side). Keep your head steady; sense rhythm, tempo, timing; and feel the torque (coil) being created between lower body and upper body as hip turn, shoulder turn, and shoulder tilt are made.
- *Finish the backswing.* There is no hurry. Smoothly transition at top of back swing, and do not rush the forward swing. Flowing energy will accumulate prior to impact.
- *Stay down with the ball.* Hit through the ball to the target.

- *Have rituals.* Prepare them for at-will relaxed focus and squeezed triggers for three types of shots.
- *Develop self-restraint and a learning response to errant shots.*
- *Know club distances.*

Four Noble Truths[53] of Golf Swing

1. We *suffer* from distance and direction issues with our golf swing.
2. We learn to use the five ball-flight laws to read ball flights and determine the causes of our distance and direction problems.
3. We learn to use the fourteen principles to *solve* our distance and direction issues.
4. We mentally rehearse and visualize; and we go to the range and the course and *practice, practice, practice* carefully selected principles to grow and develop awareness to correct distance and direction issues.

Simply Golf

- Have a warm-up process to use before you play and before each shot.
- Be a master green reader. Developing this skill is simply growing and nurturing touch, feel, and awareness.
- Hit fairways and greens in regulation. Make ups and downs and drain putts.
- Read ball flights, make corrections with principles, and practice working the ball like Bubba Watson does—deliberate fades and draws as on-the-course situations demand.
- Use tailored preshot routines for each element of the game—putting, short game, scoring wedges, and power game.
- Enjoy golf and be grateful for the gift of life.

Golf mirrors life, and it offers a tremendous opportunity to learn some of life's curriculum upon a field of friendly competition. General Douglas MacArthur, in the context of football, once remarked, "Upon the fields of friendly strife are sown the seeds that at other times and in other places, bear the seeds of victory." It is not possible to hide on-the-course—one shows up as one shows up in life.

Masters of one art have mastered all because they have mastered themselves. Each one of us is a visitor to this planet. No greater folly than to spend this short time lonely, unhappy, stressed, and in conflict with fellow visitors. Far better is to use the short time in pursuing a meaningful life, enriched by a sense of

---

[53] Ringu Tulku, 21–54.

connection with and service toward others.[54] Tolstoy comments in his diary, "We are born to die. Therefore, get it right while dying."[55] Whether on-the-course or off-the-course, Jordan Peterson's twelve rules[56] are a nice place to end and start.

- Stand up straight with your shoulders back.
- Treat yourself like someone you are responsible for helping.
- Make friends with people who want the best for you.
- Do not let your children do anything that makes you dislike them.
- Set your house in perfect order before you criticize the world.
- Pursue what is meaningful (not what is expedient).
- Tell the truth or, at least, don't lie.
- Assume that the person you are listening to might know something you don't.
- Be precise in your speech.
- Do not bother children when they are skateboarding (golfing).
- Compare yourself with where you are, not where others are.
- Pet a cat when you encounter one on the street. Dogs are OK too.

Wilber, Morelli, Leonard, and Patten offer, "No matter what-*if we don't accept every card in our hand, we can't play our best*...The deep game is not about being dealt a better hand, but about playing the cards we're dealt with as much intelligence, care, and creativity as we possibly can."[57] Awareness differentiates winners from losers—*I am silent self alone and have mastered perfect response*. Golfing enlightenment is simply playing a ball with a club from the teeing ground into the hole by fewest successive strokes "...to liberate that glorious as-yet unmanifest evolutionary potential."[58] Hit 'em high and straight, and do not miss three-foot putts.

It has been tough for the author to accept that we each are the author of our emotional experiences[59] and that a happy life beckons, acknowledging reflections of the world[60]—this is what we are and certainly is an ongoing, evolving challenge, opportunity, and journey. Accepting that life is imperfect is difficult for this perfectionist, and golf's frequent reminder is that everything is OK the way it is. As Forman notes, "One develops by working through, honestly and fully, the

---

[54]   Dali Lama, 188.
[55]   Christian and Tolstoy, 62.
[56]   Peterson, J. 2018. *12 Rules for Life*. New York, NY: Random House.
[57]   Wilber *et al*, 375.
[58]   Cohen, 159.
[59]   Nelson, 284.
[60]   Brown, 142.

demands of life as it appears right now."[61] GOLF is an AWESOME GURU!
Simple is good: go to the breath, smile, relax, focus, and trust the subconscious...

> As long as space exists
> and as long as beings endure,
> may I too remain
> to dispel the misery of the world.[62]

---

[61]   Forman, 57.
[62]   Tulku, 10.

Appendix A

Sample Vision, Current Reality Assessment, and Objectives

Strategic Objective

To model the way, on-the-course and off-the-course, of evolutionary enlightenment (where change, transition, creative friction, and evolutionary tension are the norm) and consciousness beyond ego and evolution of culture (wake up and grow up); and to come together with others in an egoless culture, free from the usual obstructions to higher creative potentials and capacities.

Strategies

- Meditation—silent self alone.
- Commit to own core values, guiding principles, ethics, morals, and evolutionary impulse.
- 100 percent responsibility—*Life happens because of me not to me.*
- Face everything, avoid nothing.
- Nurture process perspective.
- Walk the talk of cosmic conscience as a person, in relationships, and by helping others.

Vision

"Angels dancing in the cavity backs of my irons."

Goals

1. To enjoy the walk and listen to and receive infinite free messages.
2. To learn, practice, play, celebrate, relax, and activate new and higher potentials.
3. To master the technical and mental games.
4. To hit the sweet spot to unleash the club-ball sound and see the float of the ball.
5. 18-hole score (par 72): 77.
6. USGA Handicap Index: 5.

Current issues: push right and pull left, clubface not square at impact, and multiple swing thoughts (busy mind).

Objectives

➤ On every shot, deliberately quiet the mind. Let go of aversions and attachments and experience total presence, the moment in time when the mind is focused on what it is doing without the burden of extraneous thought or judgment or even labeling of whatever it is you are doing.
➤ Hit fairways: 100 percent accuracy. Current: 48 percent, miss right.
➤ Greens in Regulation: 100 percent accuracy and distance. Current: 24 percent, miss right and left, short (5–9irons, hybrid, 5FW, 3FW).
➤ Make ups and downs: 100 percent. Current: 43 percent, miss right, long and short (chip, pitch, sand, bump and run).
➤ Less than two putts per green: lag putting and putting. Current: 1.5 putts/green.

APPENDIX B

Left-Handed Golfer—Nine Ball-Flight Laws

1. *Push-draw* (inside-out, clubface closed). Ball flies straight but to left of target and then bends-draws-hooks to right.
2. *Push* (inside-out, clubface square). Ball flies straight but to left of target.
3. *Push-fade* (inside-out, clubface open). Ball flies straight but to left of target and then bends-fades-slices to left.
4. *Straight-draw* (straight, clubface closed). Ball starts straight and then bends-draws-hooks right.
5. *Straight* (straight, clubface square). Ball is on target.
6. *Straight-fade* (straight, clubface open). Ball starts straight and then bends-fades-slices left.
7. *Pull-draw* (outside-in, clubface closed). Ball flies straight but right of target and then bends-draws-hooks to right.
8. *Pull* (outside-in, clubface square). Ball flies straight and but right of target.
9. *Pull-fade* (outside-in, clubface open). Ball flies straight but right of target but then bends-fades-slices to left.

Appendix C

Club Mechanics, Body Mechanics, Ball Positions, Routine, and Ritual[63]

The purpose of this section is to offer fundamentals for putting, short game (chipping, pitching, and sand play), scoring wedges (30–110 yards), and the power game clubs—long irons, hybrids, fairway woods, and the driver. For each part of the game, five basics will be noted—club mechanics, body mechanics, ball position, routine, and ritual. Here are some definitions:

- *Club mechanics.* Physical motion and sensed physical phenomena of *club's grip, shaft, and clubhead.*
- *Body mechanics.* Physical motion of *swing* that creates clubhead speed, face angle at impact, flight pattern, carry distance, trajectory, and backspin.
- *Ball position.* Ball placement that optimizes club and body mechanics for type of shot-stroke.
- *Routine.* The sequence of actions—lasting less than eight seconds—performed in preparing to execute a shot-stroke.
- *Ritual.* Unique, consistent, relaxed focus process that immediately precedes pulling the trigger for the shot-stroke.

Putting

Putting is about direction, distance (speed), and stroke and contributes 40–45 percent of the shots made during a conventional round of eighteen holes.

---

[63] The fundamentals are explained for a right-handed golfer. Changes for a left-handed golfer are noted in parentheses (LH…).

- Club Mechanics

  The goal of putting mechanics is to have control of the ball's speed and direction. There are generally three requirements for a putter to get the ball in the hole: clubface alignment, the path of the club, and contact of the clubface with the ball. At impact (1) the clubface must be perpendicular to the desired ball-target line; (2) the path of the club should feel natural and free, be pendulum-like, and/or replicate a swinging screen door; and (3) the contact of the sweet spot of the clubface must be through the ball and strike the equator of the ball.

- Body Mechanics
  - Set-up (GASP)
    - ✓ *Grip.* Both hands feel as a single unit—not too loose, not too tight; palm of right hand (LH golfer: palm of left hand) and back of left hand (LH golfer: back of right hand) face target and are parallel.
    - ✓ *Aim.* Aim is critical, parallel left (LH golfer: parallel right) of ball-target line.
    - ✓ *Stance.* Feet a comfortable distance apart, 14"-16". Feel static balance; toes and heels should not be able to leave the ground.
    - ✓ *Posture.* T-cubed—*turn* forearms, *tuck* elbows, and *tilt* spine forward for comfort.[64]
  - Swing Motion
    - ✓ *Single lever.* With good set-up posture, the "left shoulder–right shoulder–arms–hands–grip–putter" move as a coordinated triangle that pivots at the swing point just above the breastbone.
    - ✓ *Triangle awareness.* Upper arms swing free of sides of upper torso; sense the free and natural pendulum or flowing screen-door path and feel the smooth, silky motion.
- *Ball position.* Experiment starting with one ball forward of center of stance. Note: consider marking the diameter of the ball with a line to facilitate putter face aim and alignment with ball-target line.
- *Routine.*
  - Read the green with horizontal, "binocular-like vision" that will program the subconscious to deliver the right direction and speed.
  - Visualize the shot required.
  - Make rehearsal strokes as necessary. Rehearsal strokes warm up and text the subconscious to energize the trained muscles to produce the desired results.

---

[64] Todd Sones, Coutour Golf.

44

o   Sense touch and feel. Touch programs the subconscious for the "what" direction and speed are required for the putt. Feel subconsciously senses "how" muscles will produce the required putt.

o   Move to ball and set up: eyes over ball, back hand swings freely to presented putter grip, feel static balance at body center. Tilt forward on toes and backward on heels and from side of left foot to side of right foot, sensing that the toes and heels and sides of the feet are not able to leave the ground. Release detected tension.

- *Ritual.*
o   Relaxed focus and squeeze the trigger.

Short Game

The short game and putting account for *60–65 percent of the shots* made during a conventional round of eighteen holes of golf—a very clear message about study, reflection, and practice priorities. The short game consists of chipping, pitching, and sand shots. The goal is to save putts by either putting the ball in the hole or placing shots in a three-six foot circle around the hole. Knowing distances for various short game clubs is critical for short game success and improved scoring.

- Chipping
  Chipping is used for shots off the green and normally twenty or fewer yards from the hole. The golfer normally chooses to chip the ball when putting is not possible.
  o   Club Mechanics
    ✓   *Single-lever swing motion.*
    ✓   *Triangle.* Left shoulder–right shoulder–hands–grip–club; be conscious of freedom of upper arms from the sides of the upper torso.
    ✓   *Club selection.* Pick a target on the green, three to four feet from the fringe; use the lowest trajectory club that will hit the target, and roll the ball to the hole. Typical clubs from which to choose are the 5, 7, or 9 irons; PW; and SW. Other clubs can be used: putter[65], hybrids, fairway woods, and GW. Practice direction, distance, and air time–roll time with your favorite clubs. Thicker grass requires higher-lofted clubs and a ball position that is back in the stance. Target for no grass between the clubface and the ball, and pay attention to the club path to ensure the clubface moves along the desired ball-target line.

---

[65]   1999. *Dave Pelz's Short Game Bible: Master the Finesse Swing and Lower Your Score.* New York, NY: Aurum, 219-220, 8.11 "The Chiputt."

Note: Consider marking distances for short game clubs with a piece of white tape or address label below the grip on the backside of the shaft. To eliminate a swing variable, consider having wedges the same length, and mark the length of the other longer clubs used for chipping at this same length.

- o Body Mechanics
  - ✓ Set-up (GASP)
    - ➤ *Grip*. Experiment to discover what works for you. Same as putter—overlapping, interlocking, or ten-finger. Both hands should feel as a single unit—not too loose, not too tight. Palm of right hand (LH golfer: left hand) and back of left hand (LH golfer: right hand) face the target and are parallel. Wrists are cocked down to facilitate having relatively firm wrists and a steady triangle. Only toe of club touches ground. Heel of club is off the ground to prevent it from hitting the ground at impact.
    - ➤ *Aim*. Body aligned parallel left (LH golfer: parallel right) of ball-target line; clubface aligned perpendicular to ball-target line.
    - ➤ *Stance*. Feet six to eight inches apart; feel static balance.
    - ➤ *Posture*. Place 60–65 percent of weight forward on left foot (LH golfer: right foot). Note: Tip toward target after other parts of set-up are complete. Choke up on grip to point where grip meets shaft, hands in front of left thigh (LH golfer: right thigh).
  - ✓ *Swing motion*. Visualize pulling the club through with smooth, rhythmic, free arms from body motion. No flip; swing arms and club as unit. Back and forward while brushing the grass; slightly descending, crisp impact. No grass between ball and clubface hitting little ball before big ball—follow through moving straight down the line through impact and 20 percent of backswing for follow through.
- o Ball Position
  Experiment by starting with center of stance. Preference option: front of right toe (LH golfer: left toe) before opening stance 20 degrees by rotating on heels. Ball is now off of right heel (LH golfer: left heel). With the ball back, ball is long gone before a chunk can occur.
- o Routine
  - ✓ Shot required.
  - ✓ Club selection.

      ✓ Visualize shot and pick a close-in target three to four feet onto green.

      ✓ Rehearsal swings as required.

      ✓ Sense touch and feel to program the subconscious.

      ✓ Move to ball, set up, and create silent space.

  o Ritual

    Relaxed focus and squeeze the trigger. Note: eight seconds max from start of routine through ritual, relaxed focus, and squeeze of trigger.

- Pitching

Pitching is shots of thirty yards or less to the hole. The golfer normally chooses to pitch when the ball cannot be putted or chipped and/or there is an obstacle between the ball and the hole that needs to be negotiated with a shot that has high trajectory. Example: Shooting over a greenside bunker. The goal of the pitch shot is to have the ball finish inside a three to six-foot circle around the cup. Knowing club distances is critical for effective pitch shots.

  o *Club mechanics.* Club selection is based on ball-target distance. The four key club variables required to produce the desired shot are as follows:

    1. The clubface angle must be perpendicular to the ball-target line.

    2. The club path must be parallel to the ball-target line.

    3. Contact with the ball needs to be centered on the clubface.

    4. The angle of attack needs to ensure that the golf ball is struck before the ground is struck and the divot is created. Remember little ball first and hit down to hit up.

  o *Body mechanics.*

    ✓ Set-up (80-85 percent of effective shot)

      ➢ *Grip.* Neutral

      ➢ *Aim.* Parallel left (LH golfer: parallel right); intermediate target; align clubface then align feet; open left foot (LH golfer: right foot) 30 degrees.

      ➢ *Stance.* Heels twelve to fourteen inches apart. Feel static balance. Feel and release tension.

      ➢ *Posture.* Relaxed, free of tension.

    ✓ Swing motion

    Synchronized, finesse swing.[66] Hips follow shoulders. Smooth, dead hands swing. Clock System[67] for controlling distances with the back swing. Takeaway is critical. Follow through to show

---

[66] *Dave Pelz's Short Game Bible*, 62–78.

[67] *Ibid.*, 62–78.

heel of right foot (LH golfer: left foot). Club over left shoulder (LH golfer: right shoulder). Finesse swing is upper body, no torque. Lower body follows shoulders. Feel dynamic balance, timing, tempo, and rhythm and feel and release tension. Note: Clock System. See *Dave Pelz's Short Game Bible,* pages 62–78. Each wedge is marked with white tape or address label on back of shaft below grip shaft with six finely tuned distances: 7:30, 9:00, and 10:30 for normal grip finesse swing; and 7:30, 9:00, and 10:30 finesse swing when club is gripped where lower end of grip meets the shaft. Consider creating an Excel worksheet to maintain and/or change these distances as fine-tuning progresses, as distances change, or when new clubs arrive in the bag.

- o *Ball position.* Centered between heels. Note: error toward right heel (LH golfers: left heel) not more than one ball.
- o *Routine.* Visualize shot; select club; practice swings, as desired; select a close-in target, move to ball, and create silent space.
- o *Ritual.* Relaxed focus and squeeze the trigger.
- Sand Shots
  - o *Club mechanics.* Do not limit sand shot club selection to the sand wedge. Distance control is driven by the club selected. Use all irons and know their respective distances from greenside bunkers and fairway bunkers. Fairway bunker shots require that the ball be placed back in the stance to help insure the club strikes the golf ball before it hits the sand. Placing the ball back in the stance requires selecting a club of greater loft because the club is delofted when the ball is placed back in the stance. Because the ball is back in the stance, take a couple of practice swings to help insure the clubface follows the desired ball-target line. For green-side bunker shots, the clubface is open to 45 degrees measured from the ball-target line, and normally the club grooves follow a line drawn from the ball-target line to front of the left foot (LH golfers: right foot).
  - o *Body mechanics.*
    - ✓ Set-up
      - ➢ *Grip.* Neutral.
      - ➢ *Aim.* Left of target two to three paces (LH golfers: two to three paces right of target). Experiment with this aim point, and make calibrations as necessary.
      - ➢ *Stance.* Anchored, open stance; feet fourteen to eighteen inches apart.
      - ➢ *Posture.* Relaxed, free of tension; 60 percent of weight on left leg (LH golfer: right leg). Tilt toward target when ready.

✓ Swing Motion

All greenside bunker shots are made with the nine o'clock finesse swing because the desired distance is established by the club selected. Fairway bunker shots require a full swing, and for these shots, it is critical to square the clubface to the ball-target line before takeaway.

o *Ball position.* Forward off inside of left heel (LH golfers: right heel) for greenside bunkers; back in stance for fairway bunker shots. For greenside bunkers, the club enters the sand at the low point of the finesse swing. Experiment with one, two, or three inches behind the ball. This entry point will differ based on the texture of the sand (wet, dry, fluffy, deep, *et al.*).

o *Routine.* Visualize shot. Select club. Practice swings as desired. Select target on the green and in the sand. Move to ball and create silent space.

o *Ritual.* Relaxed focus and and squeeze the trigger.

Scoring Wedges

Scoring wedge shots are those shots of thirty to one hundred yards from the hole. Knowing the respective club distances is critical to an effective scoring wedge shot. The goal of a scoring wedge shot is to have the ball finish inside a six-foot circle around the cup.

• Club Mechanics: Club selection is based on ball-target distance. The four key club variables required to produce the desired shot are as follows: (1) the clubface angle must be perpendicular to the ball-target line, (2) the club path must be parallel to the ball-target line, (3) contact with the ball needs to be centered on the clubface, and (4) the angle of attack needs to ensure that the golf ball is struck before the ground is struck and the divot is created.

• Body Mechanics

o Set-up (80–85 percent of an effective shot)

✓ Grip: Neutral

✓ Aim: Parallel left (LH golfer: parallel right). Intermediate target. Align clubface then align feet. Open left foot 30 degrees (LH golfer: open right foot 30 degrees).

✓ Stance: Heels twelve to fourteen inches apart. Feel static balance. Feel and release tension.

✓ Posture: Relaxed, free of tension.

- o Swing Motion: Synchronized, finesse swing. Hips follow shoulders. Smooth, dead hands swing. Takeaway is critical. Follow through to a high finish. Show heel of right foot (LH golfers: heel of left foot) and finish with club over left shoulder (LH golfers: right shoulder). Finesse swing is upper body, no torque. Lower body follows shoulders. Feel dynamic balance—timing, tempo, and rhythm. Feel and release tension. Remember to maintain a wide arc with the left arm (LH golfers: right arm).
- Ball Position: Centered between heels. Note: Error toward right heel (LH golfers: left heel), not more than one ball.
- Routine: Visualize shot. Select club. Practice swings as desired. Select a close-in target. Move to ball and create silent space.
- Ritual: Relaxed focus and squeeze the trigger.

Full Swing

A full swing is normally used for the driver, fairway woods, hybrids, long irons, and scoring wedges when a full swing distance is required for a shot. The full swing has the following components: takeaway, back swing, transition, forward swing, impact, and follow through.

- *Club mechanics*. Club selection is based on ball-target distance. The four, key club variables required to produce an ideal desired shot are as follows:
  1. The clubface angle must be perpendicular to the ball-target line.
  2. The club path must be parallel to the ball-target line.
  3. Contact with the ball needs to be centered on the clubface.
  4. The angle of attack needs to ensure that the ball is struck before the ground is struck and a divot is created. The angle of attack for a driver will normally be ascending at impact.
- *Body mechanics.*
  - o Set-up
    Be consistent, stable, centered, and free of tension. Be aware of and feel static balance. Detect and release tension.
    - ✓ *Grip*. It should be comfortable. Grip must return clubface square to the ball. Grip is open, closed, or neutral. Left hand (LH golfers: right hand) placed on the club so that the shaft is pressed up under the muscular pad of the heel and also lies across the top joint of the forefinger. The main pressure points are the last three fingers and the heel pad. The V created by the thumb and index finger should point to the right eye (LH golfers: left eye). Right hand (LH golfer: left hand), a finger grip. The shaft

should lie across the top joint of the fingers, definitely below the palm. The two middle fingers apply most of the pressure. Practice with the thumb and the forefinger off the shaft. The V of the right hand (LH golfers: V of the left hand) points directly to the chin. Both hands should work together as one unit. The little finger of the right hand (LH golfers: left hand) locks into the groove between the forefinger and big finger of the left hand (LH golfer: right hand). The left thumb (LH golfers: right thumb) should fit snugly into the cup of the right palm (LH golfers: left palm). Experiment with various styles of the grip, and choose a grip that works for you.

✓ *Aim.* Body aligned parallel left (LH golfers: parallel right) of ball-target line.

✓ *Stance.* Comfortable, approximately shoulder width apart.

✓ *Posture.* Forward tilt—comfortable and allows full shoulder turn (coil) and shoulder tilt.

o Swing Motion

Anchored right side (LH golfer: anchored left side) with full shoulder turn (coil) and shoulder tilt. Swing back, make a smooth transition, swing through, and stay down with and through the ball. Attack the ball at impact—divot in front of the ball. Maintain width of arc and tempo, target for vertical stability of the swing center and make a full follow through. Be centered and feel dynamic balance and maintain relative stability of lower body. Have coordinated movement during takeaway and coordinated transition from backswing to downswing, target for consistent timing, tempo, and rhythm.

✓ *Takeaway.* Smooth and fluid. Swing away from ball. One piece, coordinated movement of hands, wrists, arms, feet, knees, legs, hips, and shoulders.

✓ *Backswing.* Turn shoulders (approximately 90 degrees) and hips (approximately 45 degrees). Upper body motion is around the axis of the spine. The shoulders tilt, and target to keep a flexed right knee (LH golfer: left knee) throughout the backswing. This permits windup, resistance, and transition into forward swing for release of full power at impact. Target for a stable lower body, firmly planted feet, and a relatively stable swing center. There is no hurry in completing the backswing. It is more important to have the club in proper position at the top of the backswing than to be in a hurry to put the club at the top of the swing.

✓ *Forward swing.* As the back swing is nearing completion, delay your forward arm and hand swing while initiating the transition to the forward swing by turning, moving the left hip and knees to the left (LH golfer: right hip and knees to right) toward the ball. Weight shifts to left foot (LH golfers: right foot). The torso and shoulders resist as the arms and hands are pulled down by the legs, hips, and back inside the ball-target line. Target for coordination of body and club mechanics while sensing and maintaining dynamic balance—this equates to timing.

- *Ball position.* Varies by club. Tee the driver off the inside of the left foot (LH golfer: right foot). Fairway woods and longer irons forward of center. Hybrids and shorter irons toward center of stance. Experiment with ball position to discover what works for you.
- *Routine.* Visualize shot, practice swings as desired, select a close-in target, move to ball, and create silent space.
- *Ritual.* Relaxed focus and squeeze the trigger.

Appendix D

Green Reading and Putting
Preshot Routine and Ritual

Green Reading

Every putt is a new experience and an opportunity to awaken and grow awareness. Dave Pelz notes, "If you understand more and better interpret the meaning of what your eyeballs take in from the greens, the more and better you can see the true break in putting."[68] The skill of green reading is nurturing awareness to make predictions for optimum ball tracks that will find the hole. As you place a ball marker behind the ball, a personal checklist, created from the technical genius found in *Dave Pelz's Putting Bible*, is as follows:

1. Move to a location at the *side of the hole* that permits visual examination within the six foot diameter around the hole. Look for the pure downhill direction in this circle and scrutinize the "lumpy donut" area uncovering potential footprints to be negotiated, noting any uphill in the donut hole and fixing any optimum ball track issues.
2. Stand *behind the hole* on the extended ball-hole line and verify the downhill direction.
3. Stand *behind the ball* on the ball-hole line and validate the downhill direction.
4. Move a *step downhill* and visualize a perfect ball track rolling into the hole. Sense the amount of visible break on the ball track and make a mental note of the visible break apex distance.

---

[68] Pelz, 334.

5. Visually move the visible break apex distance out to the hole; multiply it by three to establish the true break distance point. NOTE: Have experienced the "multiply by three" changes with green speed.

6. Position yourself—move downhill—until you are on the optimum true break point distance line and you can sense the true break ball track at the optimum seventeen inches past the hole speed.

7. Align line-marked golf ball with the sensed optimum true break point distance line. You are now ready to pick up your ball marker and finish the putting preshot routine.[69]

Preshot Routine

- Stand behind the ball on the ball-target line and make practice strokes to subconsciously program the stroke necessary to move the ball to the hole.
- Walk to the ball along the optimum, true break, ball-target line, mentally embracing the putter, the optimum stroke, the hole, and the ball rattling the bottom of the cup.
- Go to the breath[70] to activate awareness—focus on the in-out breath and begin to quiet the mind and release tension. As deliberate, deep breathing continues, SMILE and complete set-up:
  - ➤ *Grip.* Hands act as a single unit, not too loose and not too tight.
  - ➤ *Aim.* Parallel flow lines[71] of feet, knees, hips, forearms, and shoulders are aligned parallel with optimum true break, ball-target line.
  - ➤ *Set up.* Fine-tune ball position with eyes over ball. Check for square clubface, comfortable stance, and relaxed posture. Dance to feel static and dynamic balance. Eyes over ball; and deliberately free swing the right arm, moving putter to hands. You are now ready for your ritual.

Ritual

- *Ground.* Take a couple of deep breaths and visualize energy circulating between your feet and the earth below you. Feel static and dynamic balance, and sense a balanced, solid foundation and the environment surrounding you.

---

[69] Ibid., 339.

[70] "Holistic physicians often say that conscious breathing is the number one health practice. Spiritual teachers often call it the number one spiritual practice … the way you breathe has big effects upon your health, consciousness and well-being … Breath and feeling are inextricably linked." (Wilber, K. *Integral Life Practice*, 188).

[71] Pelz, 100.

- *Elevate.* Take three to five short, explosive breaths into the upper chest to activate the sympathetic nervous system, increase oxygen, and intensify subtle energy currents. Charge the whole body, physically and emotionally, and make a final visual touch of the target.
- *Relaxed focus.* On an out-breath, direct one-pointed concentration on the point of impact of club with ball (mindfulness). Channel all body energies into a laser beam of relaxed, focused concentration, letting go of everything (self-restraint). Sense the synchronous, flowing swing to impact with a ball creatively floating to the target (awareness).

Squeeze trigger. With absolute trust, subconsciously trigger the tension-free swing.

Recovery

Recovery restores health to the human system and can include celebrating, responding, learning, relaxing, and preliminary thoughts about the next shot. *I am centered, calm, silent, present, and at peace. My choice is to experience this moment.* Smell the roses, enjoy the day, take a deep breath, smile, and be at peace. As the period of recovery nears its end, of necessity, it includes transitioning the body and mind for that next encounter with the new canvas, your artist's tools, a golf ball, and the associated challenges of the next shot and the next moment. Every moment of life has a purpose that one can choose to embrace and energize, and in the present moment, one enjoys life and golf saturated with meaning.[72] Simply life punctuated with simple golf.

---

[72] Brown, 144.

Resources

Armour, T. 1953. *How to Play Your Best Golf All the Time*. New York, NY: Simon & Schuster.

Bhaerman, S. & Lipton, B. 2009. *Spontaneous Evolution: Our Positive Future (and a way to get there from here)*. New York, NY: Hay.

Bhodan, D. 2012. *The Lazy Man's Way to Enlightenment: What You're Looking For Is What Is Looking*. New York, NY: Right Now.

Brown, M. 2005. *The Presence Process: A Healing Journey Into Present Moment Awareness*. New York, NY: Beaufort.

Christian, R. & Tolstoy, L. 2015. *Tolstoy's Diaries Volume I: 1847-1894 (Leo Tolstoy, Diaries and Letters)*. Amazon Whispernet.

Cohen, A. 2011. *Evolutionary Enlightenment: A New Path to Spiritual Awakening*. New York, NY: Select Books.

——— 2002. *Living Enlightenment: A Call for Evolution Beyond Ego*. Lenox, MA: Moksha.

Coop, R. & Wiren, G. 1978. *The New Golf Mind*. New York, NY: Simon & Schuster.

Crittenden, J. 2010. *Golf Inc.*, "The future of golf according to Dana Garmany," Spring 2010, 28-31.

Crum, T. 1977. *Journey to Center: Lessons in Unifying Body, Mind, and Spirit*. New York, NY: Fireside.

DeVito, C. 2008. *Golf: The Players, The Tournaments, The Records*. Kennebunkport, Maine: Cider Mill Press.

DeVore, J. 2014. *Golfer's Palette: Preparing for Peak Performance*. New York, NY: Penguin.

Diaz, J. "TIGER GREAT?: Nicklaus, Player, Trevino, Miller & Faldo on going from good to transcendent." *Golf Digest*, February 2018, 59–65.

Forman, M. 2012. *A Guide to Integral Psychotherapy: Complexity, Integration, and Spirituality in Practice*. Amazon Whispernet.

Gimian, J. 2009. *Be the Change: How Meditation Can Transform You and the World*. New York, NY: Sterling.

Gallwey, W. 1998. *The Inner Game of Golf* (Revised Edition). New York, NY: Random House.

Goldstein, J. 1994. *Insight Meditation: The Practice of Freedom*. Boston, MA: Shambhala.

Golf Academy of America Teaching Manual, 2nd Edition. 2009. Chandler, AZ.

Golf Magazine, From the Editor, "Welcome to the Machine," David DeNunzio, Editor-in-Chief, August 2019.

Golf Digest, 2016, Volume 67, Number 11 A, Tribute, "Arnie: An American Legend, 1929-2016."

Golf Rules Illustrated: The United States Golf Association, An Official Publication. 2011, Hamlyn.

Hill, D. 2010. *Golf: The Players, The Tournaments, The Records*. Kennebunkport, Maine: Hallmark.

His Holiness the Dalai Lama. 2011. *Beyond Religion: Ethics for a Whole World*. Boston, MA: Houghton Mifflin Harcourt.

Jacobs, J. 1972. *Practical Golf*. Guilford, Connecticut: Lyons.

King, J. 2017. *The Heart of Golf: Assess Your Supreme Intelligence for Peak Performance*. Flat Rock, NC: Positive Mental Imagery.

Knowles, M., Holton III, E. & Swanson, R. 2014. *The Adult Learner: The definitive classic in adult education and human resource development,* 8ᵗʰ Edition, Amazon Whispernet.

Lardon, M. & Leadbetter, D. 2008. *Finding Your Zone: Ten Core Lessons for Achieving Peak Performance in Life and Sport.* New York, NY: Penguin.

Lipton, B. 2005. *The Biology of Belief.* New York, NY: Hay.

Love, D., Jr. & Toski B. 1997. *How to Feel a Real Golf Swing: Mind-Body Techniques from Two of Golf's Greatest Teachers.* New York, NY: Three Rivers.

Marriot, L. & Nilsson, P. 2001. *Play Your Best Golf Now.* New York, NY: Gotham.

Mickelson, P. 2009. *Secrets of the Short Game.* New York, NY: Harper Collins.

Millman, D. 1994. *The Inner Athlete: Realizing Your Fullest Potential.* Walpole, NH: Stillpoint.

Mitchell, S. 1988. *Tao Te Ching.* New York, NY: Harper.

Murphy, M. 1972. *Golf in the Kingdom.* New York, NY: Penguin.

Nelson, B. 2019. *The Emotion Code: How to Release Your Trapped Emotions for Abundant Health, Love, and Happiness.* New York, NY: St. Martin's Essentials.

Palmer, A. 2016. *A Life Well Played: My Stories.* New York, NY: St. Martin's.

Parent, J. 2002. *Zen Golf: Mastering the Mental Game.* New York: NY: Doubleday.

Pelz, D. 2000. *Dave Pelz's Putting Bible: The Complete Guide to Mastering the Green.* New York: NY: Doubleday.

———— 1999. *Dave Pelz's Short Game Bible: Master the Finesse Swing and Lower Your Score.* New York, NY: Aurum.

Peper, G. 1995. *The Story of Golf.* New York, NY: TV Books.

Peterson, J. 2018. *12 Rules for Life.* New York, NY: Random House.

Price, R. 2004. *The Ultimate Guide to Weight Training for Golf.* Cleveland, Ohio: Price World.

Reid, C. 2005. *Get Yourself in Golf Shape: Year-Round Drills to Build a Strong, Flexible Swing*. New York, NY: Rodale.

Ringu Tulku. 2005. *Daring Steps Toward Fearlessness*. Boulder, CO: Snow Lion.

Roberts, K. 1962. *Yoga for Golfers*. New York, NY: McGraw-Hill.

Rotella, B. 2004. *The Golfer's Mind: Play to Play Great*. New York, NY: Free Press.

———2012. *The Unstoppable Golfer: Trusting Your Mind & Your Short Game to Achieve Greatness*. New York, NY: Free Press.

Ruiz, D. 1997. *The Four Agreements: A Toltec Wisdom Book*. San Rafael, CA: Amber Allen.

Sakyong Mipham. 2003. *Turning the Mind Into an Ally*. New York, NY: Riverhead.

Schaef, A. & Fassel, D. 1988. *The Addictive Organization: Why We Overwork, Cover Up the Pieces, Please the Boss and Perpetuate*. San Francisco, CA: Harper & Row.

Shapiro, E. & Shapiro, D. 2011. *Be the Change: How Meditation Can Transform You and the World*. New York, NY: Sterling Ethos.

Shoemaker, F. 1996. *Extraordinary Golf: The Art of the Possible*. New York, NY: Pedigree.

Shoemaker, F. 2007. *Extraordinary Putting*. New York, NY: Penguin.

Thich Nhat Hanh. 2015. *Silence: The Power of Quiet in a World Full of Noise*. New York, NY: Harper One.

Tolle, E. 2005. *A New Earth: Awakening to Your Life's Purpose*. New York, NY: Plume.

——— 1999. *The Power of Now: A Guide to Spiritual Enlightenment*. Novato: CA: New World.

Toski, B. 1977. *The Touch System for Better Golf*. Norwalk, CT: Golf Digest.

Tulku, R. 2005. *Daring Steps Toward Fearlessness: The Three Vehicles of Buddhism*. Ithaca, NY: Snow Lion.

Wilber, K. 2000. *Integral Psychology: Consciousness, Spirit, Psychology, Therapy.* Boston, MA: Shambhala.

Wilber, K. *et al.* 2008. *Integral Life Practice: A 21ˢᵗ Century Blueprint for Physical Health, Emotional Balance, Mental Clarity, and Spiritual Awakening.* Boston, MA: Integral.

About the Author

John Edwin DeVore, PhD

- PhD (human communication) and MBA, University of Denver; MA (religious studies), Naropa University; BS (military art and engineering), United States Military Academy, West Point, New York; associate of business (golf management) and advanced teaching, the Golf Academy of America.
- Military service: US Army, eight years including two years of combat during the Vietnam War. Airborne School, Ranger School, well decorated, and honorably discharged as major.
- Corporate leadership and management executive and consultant for twenty-seven years.
- Publications: *Sitting in the Flames: Uncovering Fearlessness to Help Others; Golfer's Palette: Preparing for Peak Performance; Sunland Springs Golf Club Case Study: How to Buy a Golf Course;* and *Golf as Guru: Mindfulness, Awareness and Self-Restraint.*
- President and owner, Golf-Life Mastery, a golf coaching business.
- Golf, seventy-plus years.

Contact Information: email JohnDeVore@aol.com; website www.johnedwindevore.com.